Power Yoga

A Beginner's Guide

Published By Shaharm Publications

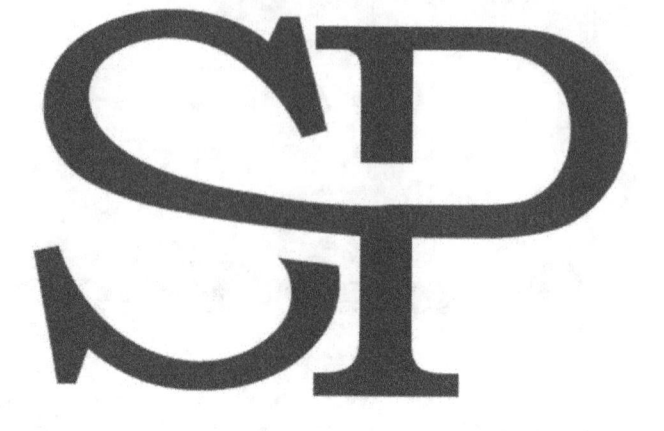

For a full list of books by Shaharm Publications, please go to:

http://www.shaharmpublications.com

Copyright © 2014-15. All rights reserved worldwide.

No part of this publication may be replicated, redistributed, or given away in any form without the prior written consent of the author/publisher.

Table of Contents

1. Introduction

Yoga is considered one of the most effective ways to reduce stress and increase a general overall feeling of happiness and contentment as well as improving flexibility and strength in the body. The common view of yoga used to be one of quiet, controlled, gentle chanting in a variety of serene poses. In the 1990s that view expanded to include power yoga - a new, more intense and energetic form of the practice, with different benefits and results. Power yoga is a westernized form of yoga that is more physically vigorous than more traditional eastern forms, with more focus on the physical demands than on the spiritual side.

What Is Power Yoga?

The practice that is now known as power yoga originates in a traditional form of yoga known as Ashtanga Vinyasa yoga or "Ashtanga yoga" for short. The "Vinyasa" part of the name refers to the breathing part of the practice. Breathing is a key element of all yoga styles, and in particular, it is a foundation of Ashtanga yoga and Power yoga. Power yoga is a variation on Ashtanga and includes the "breathing with sound" feature of the traditional Ashtanga practice. Each move in power yoga is accompanied by an inhale or exhale of breath.

The breathing is deep and audible; with practitioners making a sound as they exhale that is compared to the sound of the ocean. This intense and vocal breathing technique gives practitioners a strong point of focus that enables them to perform each move more effectively. Power yoga, unlike other forms of yoga, is fast moving, with very little time spent in any one particular pose. This variation on the Ashtanga was created in America by two American yoga teachers around the same time. One was based in New York while the other was based in Los Angeles; both had Sri K. Pattabhi Jois, a master of Ashtanga yoga.

The purpose of developing power yoga from Ashtanga was to make the practice more accessible and attractive to westerners. The idea worked, and power yoga was welcomed into the world of gym workouts and weight loss programs. The intensity of the exercises combined with the regimented breathing patterns result in an all-round conditioning of the body. The moves are designed to increase the body's internal temperature, produce sweating and increase the circulation and flow of oxygen to the organs.

2. The Differences between Yoga and Power Yoga

Although there are many different forms of yoga, power yoga is significantly different in both its practice and its benefits. The yoga that most people are familiar with is a gentle, slow practice that still has the focus on breathing, but in a very slow and calm manner. The poses are held for five breaths or more, developing endurance and flexibility in addition to a calm mind. The practice of yoga is an effective way to not only reduce the effects of stress, but, over the long-term to increase the practitioner's ability to handle stress in day-to-day life. Power yoga, while using some of the same poses as other forms of yoga, is a much more energetic and fast-paced form of the practice.

Whereas in other forms of yoga the practitioner moves very slowly from one pose to another and then holds each pose for a period of time, in power yoga the sequence of poses moves much more quickly. With the focus in power yoga on the movement rather than on holding the pose as it is in other forms of yoga, the flow is faster and getting from one pose to another is more demanding on the body. The focus on the audible breathing that accompanies each move is a way of disciplining and controlling the moves as well as the mind, and the moves are designed to develop strength and stamina as well as flexibility.

Power yoga is more flexible in the sequence of moves and poses than other forms of yoga. Ashtanga yoga, along with other forms of yoga, have a specific series of patterns and moves that are followed fairly strictly, while power yoga is more fluid and creative with the practitioners and teachers varying their choice of moves and sequences more widely. The meditative aspects of the other forms of yoga are not a part of power yoga, which is closer to a gym work out than a meditation. In fact, power yoga could be described as an aerobic yoga.

3. The Benefits of Power Yoga

Power yoga produces benefits to both the physical body and the mind. Although the focus is more on the physical, the mental benefits are still substantial, and it provides a more holistic experience than many regular types of aerobic exercise.

Physical Benefits

The physically demanding routines increase flexibility as other forms of yoga do; however in addition to this, power yoga is particularly effective for increasing strength and stamina as well. With its low impact activity, power yoga is gentler on the body than many other types of exercise, and this also means it is accessible by a larger number of people. Those who are unable to take part in other intensive activities such as weight lifting and sprinting will be able to benefit from power yoga. It can be adjusted in various ways to suit the individual; and in fact there are specific routines for pregnant women, children and elderly people.

Power yoga is a highly effective way of strengthening the bones and preventing osteoporosis. It achieves the same effects in this area as those gained from weight training, but with less strain on the body. It also boosts the immune system by increasing the drainage of lymph, which helps the lymphatic system to more effectively fight infections and diseases. The lymphatic system is responsible for killing cancerous cells as well as disposing of toxins from the body. Increasing the lymph drainage increases the efficiency and potency of these processes.

This form of yoga, along with other yoga practices, results in a reduction of clot-promoting proteins by reducing the stickiness of platelets. This means thinner blood, which can help to lower the risk of clots that cause strokes and heart attacks. In addition to strengthening the bones and ligaments, yoga helps to strengthen the back and spine, resulting in a reduction of back pain as well as a lower risk of injury. The practice of power yoga has a positive effect on the posture of the body, correcting alignment that may be causing a variety of physical problems as well as aiding digestion and various other functions within the body.

Power yoga is an effective form of exercise for weight loss since it burns more calories than regular yoga and builds lean muscle mass. The increase of lean muscle mass results in an increase in the resting metabolic rate which means the body will be burning more calories while at rest due to the fact that muscle takes more energy to maintain than other tissues. The strengthening of muscles, bones and ligaments that is achieved through power yoga also helps to prevent injuries from other physical activities.

Mental Benefits

In addition to the significant physical benefits from practicing power yoga, the mental benefits are impressive and substantial as well. As is the case with other forms of yoga, the effects on stress management are exceptionally high. Those who practice yoga have been found to produce lower amounts of stress chemicals, enabling them to handle stress more effectively as well as decreasing the effects of stress on the body and mind. Power yoga also increases the production and absorption of "feel good" chemicals in the brain.

Practitioners of power yoga experience an increase in memory ability and the ability to concentrate and focus. Although other cardiovascular activity has a positive effect on both concentration and memory as well, power yoga has been shown to be even more effective than other cardio activities. Power yoga has been found to improve the self-image and body image of those who practice it regularly. In fact, studies of women who take part in other aerobic activity and women who practice power yoga have shown that, although both groups were fit and healthy, those who practiced power yoga had a higher rate of satisfaction and appreciation for their physical state and body image.

For those who suffer from insomnia, power yoga is one of the most powerful and effective ways to improve not only the length of time it takes to fall asleep and the length of time spent asleep, but also the quality of sleep. Those who practice power yoga enjoy deeper, more restorative and rejuvenating sleep than those who do not take part in the activity.

Overall, the combination of physical, mental and emotional benefits from regularly practicing power yoga make it an effective way to improve quality of life as well as physical fitness and weight loss or weight maintenance. In addition to the direct benefits that can be gained from practicing power yoga, the knock-on effects are varied and far-reaching. The results of feeling physically, mentally and emotionally stronger and more energized can result in, an increase of productivity in the work place as well as the domestic environment; improved relationships and communication in both work and social situations; clearer and more positive thought processes; a better ability to make decisions and take advantage of opportunities; stronger support with friends and family; healthier choices in lifestyle and diet; and many more.

4. The Importance of Breathing in Power Yoga

All forms of yoga have a strong focus on breathing and breath control; it is one of the foundations of effective yoga practice. In power yoga, it is used as a link between poses and a source of the power that fuels the movement from one pose to another. All breathing in power yoga is done only through the nose - both inhaling and exhaling. Breathing through the nose is the most efficient way to get oxygen from the breath into the lungs and then in turn, into the blood stream, which delivers it to the cells.

Breathing in through the nose is universally accepted as healthier than breathing in through the mouth for two main reasons:

- The nose is lined with tiny hairs called cilia that filter impurities from the air inhaled as it enters the body. This helps to protect the lungs and the rest of the body from a wide variety of unwanted particles

- The nose provides the first "treatment" of the air coming into the body by warming air that is cold, and cooling air that is too warm

Although teachers of many forms of exercise, including dance, martial arts and aerobics teach students to inhale through the nose and exhale through the mouth, exhaling through the nose gives the body a second opportunity to retrieve oxygen from the out breath. This means more oxygen for the body for every breath inhaled and exhaled. Exhaling through the nose means the lungs are working more efficiently and effectively.

Apart from ensuring that the body is receiving plenty of oxygen during the exercise, the breathing in power yoga also provides an important point of focus. By concentrating fully on the breath going in and the breath going out, the practitioner is able to remain fully focused and in the moment; which allows for more effective practice. The breaths are deep, controlled and steady with specific points for inhaling and exhaling.

The type of nose breathing that is used for power yoga is called ujjayi or "ocean breath". The description "ocean breath" refers to the sound made during both inhaling and exhaling. It is produced by breathing deeply in the throat rather than just sniffing through the nose. Think "Darth Vader"! If you take a moment to breathe in and out through your nose, slightly constricting the back of your throat, and pulling the air through it, and making the sound of a "heavy breather" or Darth Vader, you will find the right technique. These are long, slow, deep breaths in and out.

This ocean breath style of breathing increases the body's internal heat and helps to purify the body. In addition to this, the fact that the breath is audible means that it provides a strong point of distraction for the conscious mind. By listening to your "Darth Vader" breathing, your mind will be distracted from thinking of anything outside of the moment. This means you leave all worries and concerns outside of the class; it also helps to prevent any negative thoughts about the exercise itself. With the audible breath pulling your mind's focus, you are able to perform a far more effective power yoga session.

Generally speaking, in power yoga you will be breathing out as you move into a posture, and then inhaling as you move out of that posture. Unlike other forms of yoga, in power yoga very little time is spent holding each pose, this means the movement is constant and fluid; and the breathing is therefore constant and fluid to match it. There are some occasions where a posture is held for a short period of time; and this is usually timed by breaths - for example, holding the posture for five breaths will mean you are holding that position while continuing to breathe in and out at the same pace you have been breathing while moving, before then moving again to the next position.

Throughout power yoga routines you will find that you will be breathing in whenever you are going against gravity and breathing out whenever you are going with gravity. As you breathe in deeply through your nose, creating slight friction at the back of your throat by closing it off slightly and creating the sound of the ocean breath (or Darth Vader), fill your diaphragm from the bottom and allow your chest to expand as you breathe in at a steady, slow pace. Breathing slowly lowers the heart rate and enables the lungs to absorb more of the oxygen from the air you inhale.

On the exhale, allow the air to escape at a slow and steady pace through your nose, again through the slight restriction in your throat that creates the whooshing sound, and allow your chest to contract as the air leaves through your nose. It is a good idea to spend a bit of time practicing this form of breathing outside of the yoga sessions so that you can become comfortable with it. Becoming comfortable with the ujjayi breath way of breathing will give you a head start in your power yoga sessions since it will become natural and automatic.

5. Vinyasa

Vinyasa refers to the movement between the poses in power yoga. This movement is more of a focus than the poses themselves. Whereas in other forms of yoga, the movement from one position to another is not as important as the time spent holding the posture itself, in power yoga it is this movement or vinyasa that is the primary focus and that gives power yoga its cardiovascular element.

Vinyasa are also used in other forms of yoga as a method of moving from one pose to another, and vinyasa yoga is also described as "flow yoga" because of the fluidity of the movement from one posture to the next. In vinyasa yoga, the exercise that is referred to as "going through the vinyasa" generally refers to a specific sequence of moving from the plank pose to the chaturanga position and then to the upward facing dog posture. However, in power yoga, the term vinyasa does not refer to any specific routine and instead refers simply to any movement that provides the transition from one position to the next.

Vinyasa are always accompanied by either an inhale or exhale of breath. The effectiveness of power yoga relies heavily on the synchronization of the vinyasa with the ujjayi breath (ocean breath) style of breathing. The two go hand-in-hand to provide the strength, power and focus in the practice of power yoga. Each vinyasa will always be accompanied by the same breath - in or out. For example, moving from the cobra position back into the downward dog posture, would be accompanied by an exhale of breath in the ujjayi style of breathing

6. Basic Power Yoga Poses or Asanas

Although power yoga is very flexible and the poses as well as the sequences can vary greatly depending on the teacher and the preference of the practitioner as well as the main goals for the practice, there are a few basic poses that are generally common to all power yoga sessions.

Downward Facing Dog

In this pose, your hands are placed flat on the floor at the front of the yoga mat, with your feet at the other end of the mat. Arms and legs are straight, hips lifted up high, back straight and your head in line with your spine so that you are looking towards your feet. In power yoga you will exhale getting into this position.

Upward Facing Dog

Lying flat on the yoga mat, with your hands placed flat on the mat in line with your waist; straighten your arms, lifting your chest off the floor and pushing your head back. Keep your hips and the full length of your legs on the floor as you arch your back. In power yoga you will inhale into this position.

Lunge Pose

From the downward facing dog pose, inhale as you bring your hips down and move your right foot up to place it on the inside of your right hand, lifting both hands so that the fingertips remain in contact with the mat. Keep your back straight and your head up, looking straight ahead. This is the right lunge pose, you will repeat the move using the left foot as well.

Warrior 1

From the lunge pose, lift your arms straight out to the sides, and continue lifting them up towards the ceiling until both hands are above your head with arms straight and palms together. Swivel your back foot so that it is at an angle that enables you to place it flat on the floor. Your head should be back so that you are looking at your hands. You will inhale getting into this pose in power yoga.

Warrior 2

From Warrior 1 simply lower both arms, keeping them straight and position them so that if you have your right leg forward in the lunge, your right arm is stretched out straight in front of you, over your right knee and your left arm is stretched straight out behind you, over your left leg. Your chest is opened up and you have twisted your torso so that it is aligned with your hips. In power yoga you will inhale into Warrior 2.

Reverse Warrior Pose (also known as Viparita Virabhadrasana)

From Warrior 2, drop the back arm to rest the hand on the back of the thigh of the back leg while lifting the front arm straight up to the ceiling, above your head. You will inhale into the reverse warrior.

High Plank (also known as Chaturanga Dandasana)

The high plank pose is similar to a push-up in that your weight is on your hands and toes with your hands placed approximately in line with your shoulders. You need to keep your back completely straight. You will inhale into this pose.

Low Plank

From the high plank, exhale as you bend your elbows, pushing your body forward as you lower it until the top half of your arms is parallel with the floor. Keep your head straight and in line with your spine, and your back straight with your weight supported on your hands and toes.

Sun Salutation Back Bend

This is often the first position of a power yoga session. Stand straight, with your feet together and your hands by your sides. As you inhale, lift both arms straight out to your sides, and up towards the ceiling until they are straight up above your head. Push your hips forward and arch your back and push your arms back, positioning your head back so that you are looking at your hands.

Extended Side Angle Pose

Exhale into this pose. From the lunge, lean forward and, if you have your right leg in front in the lunge, place your right hand flat on the mat next to your right foot, twisting your torso to the left and lifting your left arm straight up to the ceiling. Keep your head aligned with your spine and look up at your left hand. Do the same on the other side, with the left foot and left hand forward.

Triangle Pose

This pose is the same as the extended side angle pose except that instead of the front leg remaining bent, it is straightened with the hip belonging to the back leg pushed up and out. The arm positions and upper body position are the same, and the head is in the same position, with the visual focus on the hand that is up above the head, but both legs are now straight. You will exhale into this pose during power yoga.

Half Moon Pose

For this pose you will need to put your weight on one leg with the same side hand on the mat for balance. With your legs straight but with soft knees, place both hands on the mat in front of you. Lift your left leg straight out behind you and open up your body to the left as you lift your left arm straight up to the ceiling, following it with your eyes so that your head has turned. Keep the fingertips of your right hand spread on the mat in order to help you to keep your balance. You will inhale as you go into this pose.

Padangusthasana (also known as the Big Toe pose)

This pose can be done lying down and standing. To begin with it is best to stick to the lying down version as the standing version needs an advanced ability to balance as well as extra flexibility. Start by lying flat on your back on the mat. As you inhale, lift your right leg, keeping the knee straight, grab the big toe of your right foot with your right hand, holding the position for five ocean breaths before you let go of your toe and lower your leg back down to the floor as you exhale.

Padahastasana (also known as the hand to foot pose)

For this pose you will exhale as you move. Starting from a standing position with your back and legs straight, and your arms straight up above your head, slowly bend at your waist, keeping your head in line with your spine and your arms in position either side of your ears. Keep your back as straight as possible as you continue to fold at the waist, lowering your hands down to your toes. From this position you can pull your forehead towards your shins to feel the full stretch.

Parivrtta Parsvakonasana (also known as the revolved triangle pose)

Start by standing at top of your mat, then swing your right foot out, turning your full body to the right and place your right foot towards the other side of your mat, turning your body to the right to follow your foot. You now have your left foot behind you and your right leg in front of you. Make sure that your left foot is angled at about 45 degrees out to the side.

Put your weight into your toes to secure the stance and lift your kneecaps up. Now exhale as you bend forward over your right leg, from your hips, keeping your back straight and place the fingertips of both hands on the mat either side of your right foot. Now, lift your head and your chest up and forward slightly so that you can feel the stretch. Next, move your left hand and position it on the outside of your right foot so that your left arm is now reaching across your body. Lift your right hand, and support your weight on your left hand and foot, pushing them into the ground.

Now, begin to twist your upper body to the right, lifting your right arm straight up to the ceiling with your chest open and facing the right. Turn your head to look at your right hand. To get out of the posture, release your left hand and bring your right hand down to the ground, twisting your torso straightforward again to align with your hips, and then hinge at the hips to lift your torso up to the standing position again. Pivot to the left, and repeat the exercise on that side, placing your right hand next to your left foot, and lifting your left arm straight up to the ceiling with your torso facing to the left.

Prasarita Padottanasana

Prasarita Padottanasana is a deep forward fold pose that is very effective for stretching the hamstrings. Stand with your feet between three and four feet apart, placing your hands on your hips and turning your feet so that they are either parallel or turned in slightly. Take a deep, slow ocean breath in, and extend from your lower spine, lifting your chest up, exhale as you fold forward from your hip joints, keeping your back straight.

Keep going as low as you can get, keeping your back as straight as possible. Shift your weight forward onto the balls of your feet and place your hands on the floor. Keep your head aligned with your spine. Keep your head and neck relaxed and your shoulders open. This pose can relieve insomnia, headaches and stress in addition to stretching the hamstrings.

Parsvottanasana (also known as the pyramid pose)

Get into the same position you were in for the revolved triangle pose, with your right foot in front of you and your left foot out behind you, turned out at a 45 degree angle, and place two yoga blocks either side of your right foot. Keep your kneecaps lifted, and place your hands on your hips. Lift your chest and lengthen your spine, then, exhale and keeping your back straight, slowly fold forward from your hip joints, until your back is parallel with the floor and place your hands on the blocks.

Keeping your spine completely straight, now take your hands behind your back, and rest them on your upper back with palms together and fingers pointing towards your head. As you exhale further, gently lean further forward and keep your shoulder blades down as you allow your hands to move further up towards your head. Inhale as you slowly lift your torso back up and release your arms.

Utthita Hasta Padangusthasana

This pose is an exercise in balance and strength. Start by standing with your feet together with your hands on your waist. Transfer your weight onto your left leg, and keep your back straight and your head facing forward. Inhale as you lift your right knee up to your chest and grab hold of the shin with your right hand to hold it in place. Find a spot on the wall in front of you that you can focus on with your eyes in order to help you to balance.

It can be very difficult to find your balance when you are just beginning with this pose, so you may need to keep going back to the beginning and practicing just lifting and holding your knee to your chest in order to develop your balance before you are able to move on to the next phase of Utthita Hasta Padangusthasana. When you have your balance, grab hold of the big toe of your right foot with your right hand, and then extend your leg straight out in front of you while holding on to your big toe.

Bend the knee back to your chest again, then turn it out to the right side, turning your head to the left, and then grab hold of your big toe, and stretch your leg straight out to the side while holding on to your big toe. Let go of your toe and bend the knee again, and then turn it back to the center, then straighten your leg out in front of you and lower it to the floor.

Repeat the same with the left leg. This can be a difficult pose to begin with, but simply stretch as far as you can, and each time you do it you will find you can go a little bit further and that your balance improves the more you practice it as well. Think of it like learning to ride a bicycle - it takes a while before you are able to balance effortlessly; and the more you practice, the better you will get.

Paschimattanasana

In this pose you will be sitting flat on the floor and folding forward over your legs. As you sit on the floor, have your legs stretched straight out in front of you, and keep your hips pushed back so that your back is not rounded and you are bending at the hip joints rather than the spine. Pull your lower belly in as you lift your spine. Lift your chest up, folding at your hips and exhale as you lower your chest towards your legs.

Make sure that you keep your spine straight and your lower belly pulled in. Grab hold of your big toes with your hands, and still keeping your back straight and your belly pulled in, fold yourself lower to rest your chest on your legs. Be sure to not pull on your toes with your arms in order to force yourself down. Let your torso do the work rather than your arms.

Parivrtta Utkatasana (also known as the twisting chair pose)

From a standing position with feet together, bend your knees and push your hips back as if you are going to sit down on a chair. Keep your weight forward on the balls of your feet in order to help you to keep your balance. Lift your arms above your head, and then bring them down, bending your elbows and placing your palms together in a prayer gesture.

Keeping your palms together and your knees bent, exhale as you twist to the right and place your left elbow on the outside of your right knee. Keep your elbows spread out in the prayer position so that your right elbow is now pointed towards the ceiling and turn your head to look at it. Pull your shoulder blades in together. Now, extend your arms by keeping your elbows in place as you straighten them. Be sure to keep your shoulders down so that they do not tense up towards your ears.

If you find this pose is too difficult to begin with, you can modify it by placing your feet shoulder width apart instead of together, and then place both of your hands on your right thigh instead of placing your left elbow on your right knee. Keep the spine open and stretched, and your shoulders down, feeling the stretch. As you loosen up you will be able to do the full version.

Purvottanasana

Sit on the floor with your legs straight out in front of you and your arms behind you with your hands flat on the floor, supporting you with your fingers pointed forward and spread for maximum stability. Point your feet and place them next to each other so that your big toes are touching. Twist your legs inwards so that you are turning your knees towards each other; you should feel this rotation in your hips.

Taking the weight on your hands, and inhaling, push your hips forward and lift up, straightening your arms so that your whole body is lifted off the ground and your weight is supported on your hands and feet. Keep your lower belly pulled in, your leg muscles strong and allow your head to fall back. Exhale as you lower yourself slowly back down to the mat.

Ardha Baddha Padma Paschimottanasana (also known as the half bound lotus forward fold)

Start by sitting on the floor with your legs straight out in front of you and your back straight, with your palms flat on the floor either side of your hips for support. Slide your right foot up by bending your knee, bringing your knee up to your chest. Grab hold of your knee with your right arm to hug it close to your chest. While you are doing this, be sure that you are keeping your left leg straight and the toes of your left leg flexed back.

Next, grab hold of your right ankle and lift it to cradle your lower right leg to your chest. You will be able to lift it higher and higher as you practice and loosen up. Slowly release your leg and cross your right foot over to your left hip, allowing your right knee to relax down. If you find that your knee does not comfortably relax down, you could place a yoga block underneath it for support.

Reach around your back with your right hand to grab hold of your right foot, and then gently relax your right arm so that it puts a slight and gentle pull on your right foot. If you cannot reach your right foot with your right hand by putting it around the back, you can use a yoga strap placed around your foot and then held in your right hand to allow for the extra distance between you're hand and foot.

Once you have got to the stage where you are able to relax your knee down without the use of a yoga block and you are able to grab hold of your right foot with your right hand, you can then begin to loosen further by bending forward from the hip joints to bring your forehead towards your ankle, taking hold of the big toe of your left foot with your left hand, keeping your back straight, and keeping your right leg and foot in the half lotus position.

Trianga Mukhaikapada Paschimottanasana (also known as the one leg folded forward bend)

Start by sitting on the ground with your legs stretched straight out in front of you. Bend your right leg, bringing your foot back so that the inside of your right foot is next to your right hip, with the top of the foot flat against the floor. Your left leg should remain straight out in front of you, with the toes pointed up to the ceiling. Keep both of your sitting bones on the floor.

Bring your hands together in a prayer gesture in front of your chest and inhale as you lift your arms up above your head, keeping the palms together. Then, exhale as you fold forward from your hip joints, keeping your arms in line with your ears and straight, positioning them towards the toes of your left foot. Make sure that you keep your spine straight, lengthening it as you fold forward, so that your ribs are over your left thigh, and grab hold of the toes on your left foot with both hands.

Hold this position for five deep ocean breaths, on the fifth exhalation, round your spine, lowering your head towards your left knee. Relax the back of your left leg through the stretch. Lift your head back up and flatten your back again while still holding onto the toes of your left foot. Then, let go of the toes, release and straighten your right leg, give both legs a shake to loosen them out, and return to the sitting position, ready to begin the sequence again, this time on the other side.

Marichyasana C for Beginners

Marichyasana is a twisting pose that can be very challenging for beginners; however, there is a variation that makes it easier to achieve the pose and to develop the flexibility that will allow you to eventually achieve the full marichyasana.

Start by sitting on the floor with your back straight and your legs straight out in front of you; palms on the floor either side of your hips, and your toes pulled back so that they are pointing up to the ceiling. Bend your right knee up, bringing your right foot right up, so that your leg is as bent as far as it can be. Make sure that you have allowed about the width of one hand between your right foot and your left thigh.

Inhale as you straighten your spine, lifting it up, and then, as you exhale, slowly rotate your right thigh to bring your knee across to the left. At the same time, lift your left arm and twist your torso at the waist, positioning your left arm over your right knee so that the back of your left shoulder is against the outside of your right knee. Make sure that you do not lean back, and keep your chest close to your right thigh.

Your left arm is now wrapped over your right leg, with the palm facing up. The next step is to twist your arm, to face the palm down as you wrap it around the knee, holding it in place. Position your left hand on your left hip, with the palm facing out and the knee in the middle of the arm. As you exhale, reach around your back with your right arm, and grasp the wrist of your right arm with your left hand to hold it in position. Turn your head to look over your right shoulder. This will cause a twist and rotation in your shoulders and spine.

Standing Marichyasana

A more gentle version of the marichyasana, this is a better option for those who find the sitting marichyasana too much of a challenge. You will need a yoga block and a chair, which you will need to place next to a wall. Place the yoga block in front of the chair and have the chair with one side next to the wall, but not touching it.

Place the heel of your right foot on the yoga block and the toes of your right foot on the floor so that your foot is in the position it would be in if you were wearing high heels. Place your left foot on the seat of the chair and lift your left arm to place it on the wall with your hand straight up towards the top of the wall.

Now, as you exhale, twist to your left, bending your left arm, bringing your left hand down to around shoulder height, and reaching your right arm up and placing it on the wall. Make sure that you keep your hips straight and facing forward as you twist your upper body. Repeat on the other side.

Paripurna Navasana

Start by sitting on the floor with your legs stretched out straight in front of you, toes flexed back so that they are pointed up to the ceiling, and place your hands slightly behind you with your palms flat on the floor, and your fingers pointed forwards. Push your chest out slightly in order to open it up, and tuck your chin in slightly. Slowly begin to lean back, keeping your spine straight as you bend your knees, bringing your feet closer. Then lift your feet off the floor until your shins are parallel to the floor, using your hands for support and hold that position.

The next step is to lift your hands off the floor, and straighten your arms, stretching them out in front of you towards your feet with your fingers spread and the palms of your hands facing inwards towards your legs. Keep your shoulders back and down. It is very important to keep your spine straight, not allowing it to collapse. If you are not able to do this without your spine collapsing you could hold the backs of your knees with your hands to help you to balance and support your spine.

Hold this position for five deep ocean breaths, and then return your feet back to the floor and hug your knees in to your chest, straightening your spine. Once you find it easy to hold the position with your calves parallel to the floor you can straighten your legs to make the pose more challenging.

Adho Mukha Vrksasana (also known as the yoga handstand)

As a beginner, you will need to practice this pose in front of a wall to start with until you have been able to master your balance in the handstand. Place the front of your yoga mat against a wall, then start from the position of the downward facing dog, with your hands near the front of your mat nearest the wall, and your feet towards the other end of the mat, furthest from the wall.

Lift your weight onto the balls of your feet, bending your knees slightly and lift your head a little. As you exhale, jump both feet up to your hands, landing with your knees bent. As you inhale, straighten your legs, and then exhale as you pull your chest towards your knees. Inhale as you release your hands from the floor and drop your hips as if you are about to sit down, stretching your arms straight up above your head.

As you exhale, straighten your legs to a standing position with your feet together and bring your hands together in a prayer position in front of your chest. As you inhale again, bend your knees and sink your hips back into the chair pose. Pause in the chair pose for one full breath in and out, and then lift your left knee up towards your chest.

Now, cross your left knee over your right knee. If you need to steady yourself at this point, you can use the wall until you have developed your balance. If you're left foot will reach around the calf of your right leg, you can wrap it round. If not, just place it as far around as it will reach. Sink your hips further into the sitting position at this point. Next, wrap your arms around each other with your right arm on top of your left arm, hooking either your thumbs or palms to hold them in place.

Lift your arms up as far as they will go, pushing your forearms away and sink deeper into the sitting position. Hold this position for two, long, deep ocean breaths. At this point, sink your hips lower into the seated position and lift your arms a little higher. Then, lean forward with your arms remaining in the position they are in, and unwrap your left leg from your right and stretch it back, straight out, level with your hips and in line with your spine.

Keeping your spine straight, slowly unwrap your arms and stretch them straight back to join your left leg. Then, exhale as you bring your arms forward, and place them on the mat in front of you, keeping your left leg stretched straight back out behind you. Make sure you have left enough space between your hands and the wall.

Next, placing the weight of your body onto your hands, kick up your left foot to place it against the wall, keeping your right leg reaching forward so that your legs are split. In order to develop the ability to balance without the assistance of the wall, start to practice gaining the balance using the counter weight of your right leg. As you lower your right leg slowly, it will begin to pull your left leg off the wall.

With practice you will be able to judge the distance and balance between having your left leg on the wall, and falling forward. Hold the handstand for three deep, long ocean breaths, then lower your feet to the floor straight into the chaturanga pose which is the push-up position. Transition into the upward facing dog, and then into downward facing dog. You are now ready to begin the sequence again.

Bhujapidasana for Beginners

Bhujapidasana is a test of balance, flexibility and strength. Doing the full pose is a challenge for the beginner, but there is a variation that can help you to achieve the pose more easily in order to practice it and develop the strength, balance and flexibility that will later allow you to achieve the full pose.

Start in a squatting position with your knees completely bent and your hands on the floor in front of you, bearing your full weight. Next, reach between your legs with your right arm to place your right hand underneath the heel of your right foot. You will need to straighten your legs a little to do this. Do the same with your left hand and foot. As you do this, your right knee should be over your right shoulder and your left knee should be over your left shoulder.

Make sure that your hands are flat on the floor with the fingers spread and facing forward. Next, bend your arms as you lower your hips so that your arms are now able to hold your legs. Now, keeping your feet on the floor, shuffle them over to each other and cross one over the other. The aim now is to press into your hands in order to lift your feet off the floor and achieve the balance.

This will take practice and the more you practice it, the better you will be able to maintain your balance. As you gain your balance you can point your toes and bend your arms, leaning forward slightly. If you over balance you can place your toes on the mat to steady yourself; you can also place the top of your head on the mat if you have overbalanced by quite a lot.

To exit this pose, release your feet from each other, lean over to the right hand side and release your left leg. Move your left foot around so that your left leg is now effectively kneeling on your upper arm. Do the same with your right leg and once you have both legs kneeling on your arms, send your feet back with a jump to the other end of the mat, so that your weight is now on your toes as well as your hands and you are in a plank position. Exhale as you lower the plank to just off the floor.

Baddha Konasana

Start by sitting on the floor with both of your legs stretched out straight out in front of you. Bend the left knee out to the left, pulling your foot up towards your body with the leg turned out and the sole of your foot facing towards your right leg. Do the same with the right leg, bending the knee out to the right. Your feet should now be meeting. Make sure that your feet are matched up, heel to heel and little toe to little toe, and that the soles of both feet are facing up. You may need to use your hands to manipulate your feet into this position.

When you have your feet tucked right up close to your body, place your left thumb on the base of the big toe of your left foot, and your right thumb on the base of the big toe of your right foot, and grab hold of your feet. Pull in your belly and, keeping your spine straight, exhale as you lower your chest towards the floor. Keep your head facing up and aim to place your chin on the floor.

Upavistha Konasana

Start by sitting on the ground with your legs stretched straight out in front of you. Lean back into a lying position with your spine straight, and then lift your right leg straight up. Make sure that you are not turning it out or in, keeping it straight.

Next, place your left hand onto your left thigh, flex the toes of your right foot, and grab the big toe of your right foot with your right hand, keeping both legs straight.

Next, exhale as you lift up your head and shoulders from the floor. Pull your knee towards your forehead and hold it for five breaths before releasing your head back to the lying down position, but still holding on to the big toe of your right foot. Now move your right leg out to the side, still holding the toe and keeping both legs straight and turning your head to look over to the left.

Make sure you keep your left hand pressed down firmly on the top of your left thigh to keep your hips straight so that your left hip does not lift off the ground. Hold this position for five breaths before pulling the leg back to the center, still holding on to the big toe, and exhaling as you bring your forehead back up to your knee. Inhale as you replace your head on the floor, then exhale as you let go of your toe and allow the right leg to lower back to the floor. Repeat the exercise with the left leg.

7. Sequences for Beginners

These are the two most common sequences that are used in power yoga classes and they are the best place for beginners to start.

Sun Salutation

This is an exercise that is used for warming up the body, and is an effective way to start a power yoga session.

1. Begin by standing at the front of your yoga mat, with your feet together, legs and back straight, knees relaxed, head facing forward with your chin parallel to the floor, and your hands by your sides.

2. Inhale using the ocean breath technique as you lift your arms with the elbows straight out to the sides and continue up to above your head. Look up to the ceiling as you do this, arching your back slightly and stretching your arms up and back.

3. Release the position allowing yourself to fold forwards as you exhale using the ocean breath technique; place your hands on your calves and pull your forehead towards your shins, stretching your back and legs.

4. Place your hands on your shins and inhale as you push your head forward, lifting your head and chest so that your chest is now parallel with the floor, your arms are straight, and your hands are resting on your shins. Your legs are straight and your spine stretched.

5. Now, as you exhale, place your hands flat on the floor in front of you, and step back to place your feet towards

the back of your mat so that your legs and spine are stretched out flat, and your weight is supported on your hands and toes. This position is called the plank.

6. Inhale while holding the plank; then exhale as you bend your knees, drop them and place them on the mat; lower your chest to the mat between your hands, keeping your pelvis up and arching your back and keeping your head up with your eyes looking straight ahead. You are now still supported by your hands and toes, but your chest is resting gently on the mat, with your hips in the air.

7. Next, exhale as you drop your hips to the mat, pushing up and back with your hands, arching your back pushing your chest out into the cobra position. Reposition your feet so that the tops of your feet are now flat on the mat; the full length of both of your legs and your hips are in contact with the mat. With your head up, your chest pushed out and shoulders back, and your arms slightly bent, supporting the top half of your body, hands still flat on the mat, you are now in the cobra position.

8. Inhale as you push back on your arms, bending your knees so that you are now on your hands and knees; and exhale as you continue the motion fluidly, straighten your legs, putting your weight back onto your toes and hands with your arms and legs straight, into the downward dog position. Keep your back straight and flat, and place your head so that it is aligned with your spine and you are looking towards your shins.

Bend your knees slightly if you need to, in order to make sure that your spine is completely straight. Hold this position for the count of five deep breaths in and out. Remember to keep your breathing deep, slow and audible, using the ocean breath technique.

9. Now, as you inhale, lift your head and bring your right foot forward, placing it behind your right hand; keeping your fingertips on your mat, bring your left foot forward and place it behind your left hand straightening both legs, exhaling. Lift your head and look up, and inhale as you place both hands on your shins.

10. Exhale as you place your hands on your calves and fold from the waist, pulling your head towards your shins.

11. Inhale now as you lift your head and upper body to the standing position, raising your arms up either side of your head, straight so that your hands are reaching for the ceiling above your head. Lean back, looking up and arching your back as you did at the beginning of the sequence.

12. Exhale as you lower the arms, keeping the elbows straight, back down to your sides, with your head facing straight ahead, your back straight, and your chin parallel to the floor.

Repeat these 12 steps.

Second Sun Salutation

1. From the end position of the first sun salutation, standing straight with your hands at your sides, legs straight, feet together and head facing straight forward, inhale with a deep slow breath, then slowly exhale as you bend your knees to lower yourself to the ground so that the tips of your fingers touch the floor.

2. Inhale as you lift your arms up with the elbows straight, either side of your body, to position your hands above your head, reaching for the ceiling; lifting your head up and straightening your legs slightly.

3. Exhale as you bring your arms straight down either side to place your hands on the mat in front of your feet, folding from the waist and keeping your legs straight. Tuck your chin to your chest as you stretch into this pose.

4. Keeping your fingertips in contact with the mat, inhale as you lift your head and upper body so that your back is straight and parallel with the floor.

5. Now exhale as you place your hands flat on the mat, and jump both feet back to the other end of the mat so that you are in the push-up position with your back straight. Your head should be up; elbows bent and close in to your body, and your body should be parallel with the floor.

6. Inhale as you straighten your arms into the position of upward facing dog. Your weight should now be on your hands and toes, pushing your chest out, shoulders back with your shoulder blades pulled together and your head up. Reposition your feet so that the tops of your feet are flat on the mat and your weight is now on your hands and the tops of your feet.

7. Exhale as you push yourself back into downward facing dog with your hands remaining flat on the mat, arms straight, legs and spine straight, and your head aligned with your spine, looking towards your shins.

8. Inhale as you step your right foot forward, lifting your right hand so that your right foot takes the position of your right hand, in line with your left hand, leaving your left foot where it is at the back of the mat at this time; then stretch your arms out to either side of your body, lifting them up to the ceiling, straight above your head. You will now be in a wide lunge position. Arch your back and push your arms back with your head lifted up, to feel the full stretch.

9. Exhale as you place your hands back on the mat, step your right foot back to position it in line with your left foot; and you are back to the push up position.

10. Straighten your arms, as you inhale, lifting your head and pushing out your chest back into the upward facing dog. Reposition your feet so that the tops of your feet are on the mat, with your back arched and your head back.

11. Exhale as you lift your hips and legs off the floor, pushing your body back into downward facing dog so that your weight is being supported by your hands and toes again. Your head should be aligned with your spine so that you are looking at your shins.

12. Now bring your left foot forward as you inhale, lifting your left hand and placing your left foot in the position your left hand was, in line with your right hand. Your left foot should be flat on the mat, with your left knee bent; your right leg straight out behind you, with the toes of your right leg in contact with the mat. Now lift your arms straight out either side of your body, and up towards the ceiling so that they are straight up above your head.

13. Exhale as you lower your arms again, placing both hands flat on the mat in their previous position, and jumping or stepping both feet back to the other side of the mat so that you are back in the push-up position.

14. As you inhale, lower your hips to the floor and reposition your feet so that the tops of your feet are in contact with the mat, straightening your arms and pushing back while lifting your head.

15. Exhale as you lift your hips, pushing your arms back to transition back into the downward dog. Hold this position as you breathe deeply in the ocean breath technique five times. End on an inhale before beginning the next move with an exhale.

16. Exhale as you bend your knees, putting the weight onto your hands; then inhale as you jump your feet up to join your hands, arms and legs straight, head facing down.

17. Inhale as you lift your head up, straighten your back and keep your fingertips in contact with the mat.

18. Exhale as you place your hands flat on the floor either side of your feet, folding at the waist and pulling your forehead towards your shins and tucking your chin in towards your chest.

19. Inhale as you bend your knees and lift your head; keeping your legs slightly bent as you lift both arms, straight out to the side and continuing up to reach for the ceiling with both hands above your head.

20. Exhale as you straighten your legs and bring your arms straight down either side to rest at your sides.

Power yoga is exceptionally good for the body, keeping the organs healthy and clean as well as reducing stress and helping to gain and maintain a healthy weight. It takes persistence and consistent practice in order to build the strength, flexibility and stamina to successfully achieve all of the poses, but starting as best you can, practicing every day, and being consistent and committed will result in your not only enjoying the benefits of power yoga, but also in building up an increasing amount of strength, balance and flexibility that will allow you to achieve more challenging poses.

Power yoga combines physical fitness and peak body conditioning with emotional and mental health and is an excellent way to improve your quality of life holistically.

www.ingramcontent.com/pod-product-compliance
Lightning Source LLC
Chambersburg PA
CBHW060345290526
45791CB00004B/1543